A New Path: My Journey from Corporate into Hospice and Palliative Care Leadership

GIAM Cheong Leong

A New Path: My Journey from Corporate into Hospice and
Palliative Care Leadership

Copyright © 2024 by Giam Cheong Leong

All rights reserved. No part of this book may be used or reproduced by any means, graphic, electronic, or mechanical, including photocopying, recording, taping or by any information storage retrieval system without the written permission of the author except in the case of brief quotations embodied in critical articles and reviews.

Email to gclo520@hotmail.com for permission.

Disclaimer:
While the author and publisher have made every effort to ensure that the information in this book is correct at the time of publishing, the author and publisher do not assume otherwise and hereby disclaim any liability to any party for any loss, damage, or disruption caused by errors or omissions, whether resulting from negligence, accident, or any other cause. The opinions expressed in the book are solely those of the author and should not be taken as professional advice. The author and publisher assume no responsibility for errors or omissions or for the outcomes of decisions based on the contents of this book.

First Edition, 2024

Published in Singapore

ISBN: Paperback   9798304839181
        eBook   available on Amazon

Printed by ColourXpress Media LLP

Cover design by Mary Lyka Adajar

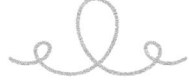

Dedicated To

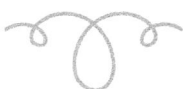

To my beloved mother, whose unwavering, selfless support continues to guide me in every endeavour I pursue. Though you are no longer with me, your love and strength remain a source of inspiration.

To my cherished mentor, Dr. Cynthia Goh, who was like a second mother to me. Together, we worked to bring comfort and dignity to those in need. Your wisdom and kindness live on in the work we did and in my heart.

To my dearest wife, who has stood by me with endless support and encouragement, helping me follow my passion for charity work. Your belief in me fuels my dedication to making a difference.

And to my three beautiful daughters — may you always strive to contribute to society with kindness, compassion, and purpose. You are my hope for the future, and I am endlessly proud of the people you are becoming.

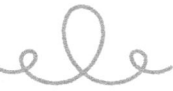

Table of Contents

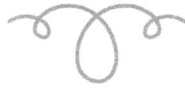

Foreword 1

Preface 3

Chapter 1: Finding Compassion – A New Beginning in the Social & Healthcare Sector 5

Chapter 2: Crafting a Vision – Aligning Corporate Skills with Compassionate Care..13

Chapter 3: Building Connections – Establishing a Supportive Care Network..21

Chapter 4: Financial Realities – Striving for Sustainability in Care 31

Chapter 5: Leading with Empathy – Shifting from Corporate to Compassionate Leadership 43

Chapter 6: Embracing Technology – Modern Tools for Patient-Centered Care 51

Table of Contents

Chapter 7: Community Engagement – The Power of Building Trust 61

Chapter 8: Navigating Compliance – Balancing Mission with Regulatory Demands 71

Chapter 9: Measuring What Matters – Assessing Impact in a Care Network 81

Chapter 10: A Look Forward – Preparing for Future Challenges and Opportunities 91

About the Author 99

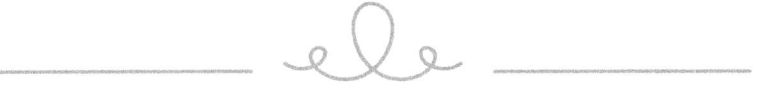

Foreword

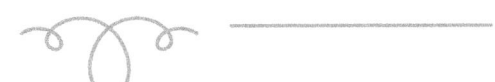

In a world where healthcare systems face mounting pressures, the need for compassionate end-of-life care defines healthcare at its best. End-of-life care is about honoring the humanity of those we care for, recognizing their unique stories, and providing a space for healing even when curing is no longer possible. My journey as a public health advocate and cancer caregiver has taught me that healthcare's greatest responsibilities are rooted in trust, love, and compassion. These values are vital, not only for those we serve but also for those who lead the systems that make health care possible. GIAM Cheong Leong's story reflects these principles and offers a powerful narrative of learning and self-realization.

Through the pages of *A New Path: My Journey into Hospice & Palliative Care Leadership*, Giam shares his experiences of moving from corporate leadership into the deeply human realm of hospice care.

Giam's journey is a reminder that leadership in healthcare is not defined by clinical expertise alone but by a compassionate heart to share the pain and listen. His reflections on bridging corporate skills with the needs of palliative care highlight the value of diverse perspectives and collaborative efforts.

It calls us to embrace the complexities of life and death with empathy, courage, and a commitment to ensure that every person receives love, care and dignity.

Dasho Dechen Wangmo

Head, Lead Agency for Mental Health (The PEMA), Royal Government of Bhutan
Founder, Bhutan Cancer Society
Former Minister of Health, Bhutan
Past President of 74th World Health Assembly

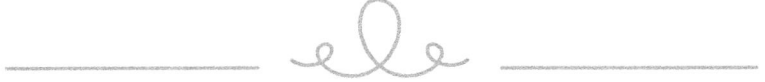

Preface

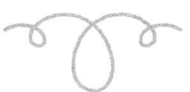

After over 20 years in corporate administration, I found myself on a transformative journey into hospice and palliative care. Driven by a deep desire to make a meaningful difference, I transitioned from strategic planning and financial metrics to the compassionate, patient-centred world of end-of-life care. Entering this field has been a profound shift — one filled with new insights, challenges, and, above all, a renewed sense of purpose. In *"A New Path"*, I share the lessons, struggles, and personal growth that have shaped my understanding of compassionate care, offering a candid look at my journey into this complex and profoundly human field.

I am, in many ways, still an amateur in this work. I continue to learn with every step, from every patient, family member, volunteer, and healthcare worker I meet. This book is not a comprehensive guide, nor does it claim to have all the answers. Rather, it is a humble sharing of what I've discovered so far — a reflection on how I've applied my corporate experience in strategic thinking, resource management, and results-driven planning to a mission of palliative and hospice care.

My hope is that this story may inspire others who are considering a similar path, especially those from corporate backgrounds who feel drawn toward a deeper, purpose-driven pursuit. There is a unique and rewarding space for those who wish to bridge the skills of the business world with the heart of social healthcare. For those who feel drawn to this mission, I warmly welcome you to reach out, connect, and explore opportunities to collaborate in charitable work.

"The New Path" is my heartfelt contribution to a world where dignity, respect, and compassion define the end-of-life journey for all. Thank you for reading, and I hope this journey offers something meaningful for you as well.

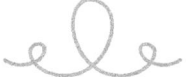

Chapter 1:
Finding Compassion – A New Beginning in the Social & Healthcare Sector

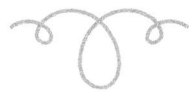

When I reflect on my journey from the structured corporate world to the compassionate, complex domain of social and healthcare sector, I am struck by how unexpectedly my path has unfolded. With over two decades of experience in corporate administration, I initially never imagined stepping into healthcare, let alone the deeply moving and often challenging field of hospice and palliative care. My transition began with an opportunity to oversee clinical operations in a community hospital, and from there, each step along the way has brought me closer to understanding the true essence of compassionate care. This chapter outlines my first encounters with palliative care, the mentors who guided me, and the profound impact it has had on me, shaping my role in advocating for equitable, sustainable care across the Asia Pacific region.

From Corporate to Clinical Operations

In my corporate life, the focus was on efficiency, strategy, and growth — a world governed by metrics and financial targets. When I transitioned to managing clinical operations in a community hospital, it was a significant shift in perspective. Suddenly, I was responsible for the smooth running of the clinical operations that catered not just to numbers but to real people in need of care. My role expanded to oversee clinical operations in a community hospital, a nursing home, a day care centre, and a chronic sick unit. This was my first immersion into a healthcare environment, and I found myself continually learning and adjusting to the unique challenges and demands of the sector.

It was during this time that I met Dr. Lee Liang Tee, a geriatrician and the hospital's medical director. Observing Dr. Lee at work was a revelation. Unlike the clinical efficiency I was accustomed to in corporate settings, Dr. Lee's approach embodied a deep sense of compassion and humanity. His commitment to integrating palliative and hospice care within the hospital was, for me, an entirely new concept. I watched as he took time with each patient, listening intently not only to their symptoms but to their fears, their hopes, and their families' concerns. His wards felt different — there was a quiet dignity in the way he cared for his patients, and an atmosphere of peace and respect permeated the space.

Dr. Lee and his team's approach was nothing short of transformative. They treated the patients with such grace, ensuring they were comfortable and that their final days were filled with as much dignity as possible. For many of these patients, their conditions could not be cured, but under Dr. Lee's care, they were made to feel valued, respected, and loved. I remember watching him speak gently with a patient's family, helping them navigate the painful reality of losing a loved one. His team provided them with emotional support, answered their questions with patience, and helped them understand the importance of a peaceful and dignified passing. This was my first true learning experience in holistic patient-centered care, and I was moved by how this approach could make such a difference to patients and their families. It was thanks to Dr. Lee that I was introduced to this world of compassionate care, a world I had previously known little about.

Tasked with Exploring Palliative Care Services

My second encounter with palliative care came when the Ministry of Health tasked the hospital administration with exploring the feasibility of building in-house palliative care services within community hospitals. It was an entirely new undertaking, and my initial focus was on logistical and operational aspects — staffing, resource allocation, and training requirements. However, as I began delving into the specifics of palliative care, I started to understand its deeper purpose.

Palliative care is not merely about managing symptoms; it's about prioritizing the quality of life, addressing emotional and spiritual needs, and supporting families through the most difficult moments. My task with the Ministry opened my eyes to the idea that care goes beyond medical interventions. I began to see that palliative care could profoundly impact both patients and their families, offering comfort, dignity, and support when it was most needed. The more I learned, the more I felt a growing conviction that this was something worth advocating for.

Stepping into Advocacy: Leading a Non-Profit in the Asia Pacific

My journey took another unexpected turn when I was offered the opportunity to lead a non-profit organization as its Executive Director, dedicated to advocating for equitable hospice and palliative care across the Asia Pacific region. This role brought me face-to-face with the vast disparities in access to quality end-of-life care across different countries. Many low- and middle-income countries struggle to provide even basic health care services, and the challenge of building sustainable models in resource-limited settings became a central focus of my work.

Stepping into this role marked the beginning of what I call my "official amateur journey" into hospice and palliative care. Despite my administrative experience, I was still very much a learner in this field. My goal was not to claim expertise but to leverage my skills and experience to support and amplify the work of those who had dedicated their lives to compassionate care. I felt an overwhelming sense of purpose, knowing that our work could make a real difference in patients' lives and provide much-needed support to their families.

Learning from a Pioneer: Professor Cynthia Goh

One of the most impactful relationships I developed during my time with the non-profit organization was with Professor Cynthia Goh, a pioneer in palliative care and one of the most selfless individuals I have ever known. Professor Goh was a highly respected palliative care physician who dedicated her life to educating healthcare professionals and advocating for palliative care in low-resource countries. Working alongside her was a privilege, and every interaction with her was a learning experience.

Professor Goh had a remarkable way of imparting knowledge. She led by example, demonstrating both the science and the art of palliative care. She believed that education was the key to addressing the over-treatment that often plagues healthcare systems, especially in resource-limited settings where patients may undergo extensive and often futile medical interventions at the end of life. Professor Goh tirelessly led volunteer teams across the Asia Pacific region, teaching local healthcare providers how to deliver palliative care that was respectful, compassionate, and culturally sensitive. Her work reminded me that hospice and palliative care are as much about the soul as they are about the body.

Thanks to Professor Goh, I learned not only the practicalities of palliative care but also its ethical and emotional dimensions. Her guidance shaped my understanding of the field, and her spirit of dedication left an indelible mark on me. Although she has since passed on, her legacy continues to inspire our work. We remain committed to carrying her vision forward, advocating for quality palliative care in communities that need it most.

A New Chapter Begins

My journey into hospice and palliative care has been, at its core, a journey of compassion. Coming from a corporate background, I initially viewed healthcare through a lens of efficiency and operations. But over the years, I've come to understand that hospice and palliative care require a different approach — one that centres on the human experience and the dignity of life. Each encounter, whether with Dr. Lee's compassionate ward management, the Ministry's mandate to explore palliative care services, or Professor Goh's dedication to underserved regions, has deepened my appreciation for the impact of this work.

I am still very much an amateur in this field, learning and growing with each new challenge. My hope is that by sharing my story, I can help others see the value of hospice and palliative care and encourage them to support its expansion. This book is not a definitive guide but rather a reflection of my experiences and insights as I navigate this complex and deeply fulfilling world.

As I embark on this journey, I carry with me the lessons I've learned from remarkable mentors, the gratitude of families we've served, and the vision of a world where every person has access to compassionate, respectful end-of-life care. This is the beginning of a new chapter in my life — one dedicated to ensuring that those facing life's final chapter can do so with dignity, comfort, and peace.

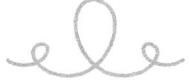

Chapter 2:
Crafting a Vision – Aligning Corporate Skills with Compassionate Care

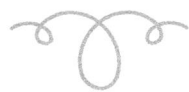

Transitioning from the corporate world to the field of hospice and palliative care was, in many ways, a transformation of purpose. My background in corporate administration had conditioned me to focus on metrics, operational efficiency, and profit margins, but the world of palliative care challenged me to see beyond numbers and outcomes. The stakes in healthcare – especially in palliative care – were not simply financial; they were profoundly human. Crafting a vision for a sustainable hospice and palliative care network meant aligning my corporate skills with the compassionate care philosophies that lie at the heart of this field.

As I stepped into my role as Executive Director of a non-profit organization dedicated to advocating for equitable hospice and palliative care across the Asia Pacific, I realized that I needed a clear vision that bridged the two worlds I had come from. The support and guidance of healthcare professionals, such as Professor Cynthia Goh and countless palliative care providers across the region, profoundly influenced my approach to this work. Each lesson learned from them shaped not only my understanding of compassionate care but also the practical steps needed to bring palliative care to communities in need.

Understanding the Importance of a Vision in Hospice & Palliative Care

In the corporate world, a vision is often about driving growth, achieving market dominance, and maximizing shareholder value. But in hospice and palliative care, a vision is rooted in compassion and service. It's about ensuring that patients and their families receive the support they need at the most challenging times of life. A vision in this field isn't merely aspirational; it's a moral commitment to provide comfort, dignity, and respect to individuals as they approach the end of life.

The task of crafting a vision for a sustainable hospice and palliative care network involved rethinking familiar corporate principles and reorienting them towards humane objectives. This vision needed to be one that balanced practical realities — such as financial sustainability and resource management — with the deeper, compassionate purpose that drives palliative care.

In my early days in this role, I turned to mentors like Professor Cynthia Goh, who had spent her life advocating for palliative care, particularly in underserved areas across Asia. Professor Goh's work exemplified the kind of vision I aspired to build. She understood that while education, advocacy, and outreach were crucial, they needed to be underpinned by a clear purpose and a commitment to sustainable impact. Her approach taught me that a vision must be firmly anchored in the needs of the community and the ethical imperative to serve with compassion.

Applying Corporate Skills to Build a Compassionate Network

One of the most significant challenges I faced was translating corporate skills — strategic planning, operational management, and resource allocation — into a framework that respected the values of hospice and palliative care. From my corporate background, I knew the importance of having a well-defined structure, clear goals, and measurable outcomes. However, I needed to adapt these tools to align with the ethos of care and empathy that underpins palliative work.

Strategic Planning with a Compassionate Lens

Strategic planning in hospice care isn't solely about setting long-term objectives; it's about crafting a vision that ensures the organization's resources, programs, and personnel are directed toward meaningful impact. Working with palliative care volunteers and teams across Asia Pacific, I learned to adopt a more inclusive approach to planning — one that involved listening to the experiences of healthcare providers, patients, and families. Professor Goh emphasized that a good plan doesn't just meet organizational targets; it must address the real, lived experiences of patients and be flexible enough to adapt to diverse needs and cultural contexts.

Through her guidance, I began to understand that a successful palliative care strategy is one that is responsive, patient-centred, and culturally sensitive. Professor Goh was known for tailoring educational programs to meet the specific needs of the communities we served. She believed that one-size-fits-all approaches were ineffective in palliative care, where personal and cultural factors are deeply entwined. Her example taught me to view strategic planning not as a rigid roadmap but as a responsive, evolving blueprint that could adapt as our understanding of each community's needs grew.

Resource Allocation and Financial Sustainability

In the corporate world, resource allocation is often about maximizing returns. In hospice and palliative care, it's about maximizing reach and impact. Financial sustainability is critical, but it must be balanced with the imperative to provide care to those in need, regardless of their financial situation. One of the challenges I faced early on was managing limited resources while ensuring that our programs reached as many people as possible, particularly in low-resource settings.

Professor Goh's approach to resource management was both pragmatic and compassionate. She was a master at doing much with little, finding innovative ways to stretch resources while maintaining the quality of care. Working alongside her, I learned the importance of prioritizing services based on community needs and leveraging local resources to extend our reach. By collaborating with local healthcare providers, training community volunteers, and partnering with local organizations, we could build a more sustainable model of care that didn't rely solely on external funding.

In addition, Professor Goh taught me that advocacy is an essential component of sustainability. By educating local leaders and policymakers about the value of palliative care, we could secure support that would help sustain our programs over the long term. This was a powerful lesson in how a well-crafted vision — one that prioritizes advocacy and community engagement — can create a ripple effect that extends beyond the organization.

Building a Culture of Compassionate Leadership

Leadership in the corporate sector often emphasizes efficiency, productivity, and growth. However, in hospice and palliative care, leadership requires a commitment to empathy, patience, and resilience. I realized that fostering a compassionate culture was as crucial as any operational strategy. A vision rooted in compassion had to be lived out not only through our programs but through the way we worked with our teams, patients, and communities.

One of the most inspiring aspects of working with Professor Goh and the healthcare providers in palliative care was witnessing their selfless dedication to their patients. Professor Goh herself exemplified compassionate and servant leadership. She didn't just instruct; she listened, supported, and encouraged everyone around her. She understood that working in palliative care was emotionally taxing and that caregivers needed empathy and encouragement to sustain their dedication.

Learning from her, I began to adopt a more supportive and inclusive leadership style. I realized that listening to the concerns of staff, acknowledging their challenges, and providing emotional support were essential aspects of fostering a compassionate work culture. Creating an environment where team members felt valued and supported not only improved morale but also reinforced our collective commitment to the vision of compassionate care.

Advocacy and Education as Pillars of a Compassionate Vision

Advocacy and education became core pillars of my vision for hospice and palliative care. The Asia Pacific region faces unique challenges, with significant disparities in access to many healthcare services. Working with healthcare providers in the region, I saw firsthand the need for targeted advocacy to increase awareness and policy support for palliative care.

Professor Goh was a tireless advocate for palliative care, particularly in low-resource settings. Her dedication to educating healthcare professionals, policymakers, and the public about the value of hospice care was transformative. Through her example, I came to understand that a sustainable vision requires not only direct service delivery but also a robust advocacy component. By raising awareness, training healthcare providers, and engaging local leaders, we could build a foundation for long-term impact.

Education was equally essential to our mission. I learned that providing high-quality care in low-resource settings required ongoing training and capacity-building. Professor Goh's commitment to education was contagious, and I found myself deeply invested in our training programs, which aimed to equip healthcare providers with the skills and knowledge to offer compassionate, culturally sensitive care. Our work in education wasn't just about imparting skills; it was about instilling the values of empathy, respect, and patient-centered care in every healthcare provider we trained.

A Vision Realized through Collaboration and Commitment

Crafting a vision for hospice and palliative care that aligns corporate skills with compassionate care principles has been both challenging and rewarding. My work with Professor Goh and the palliative care professionals across Asia Pacific has taught me that true leadership in this field requires humility, adaptability, and a deep commitment to serving others.

This vision isn't one I've created alone. It's a collective effort, built on the dedication of healthcare providers, the resilience of patients and families, and the invaluable guidance of mentors like Professor Goh. Together, we've created a foundation for palliative care that respects both practical realities and the human spirit — a vision that, I hope, will continue to bring comfort and dignity to those in need for years to come.

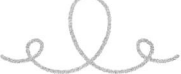

Chapter 3:
Building Connections – Establishing a Supportive Care Network

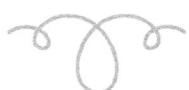

In the world of hospice and palliative care, no organization operates in isolation. Building connections and establishing a supportive care network are essential steps in providing holistic, compassionate care to patients and their families. For me, transitioning from the corporate world, where collaboration was often transactional, to the field of palliative care presented a new challenge: creating relationships rooted not in profit but in shared purpose and mutual support. This chapter delves into my journey of building a supportive care network, tapping into my own experiences, the lessons learned, and the people who have helped shape my understanding of what it truly means to work as part of a care community.

Embracing the Concept of a Supportive Network

In the corporate world, networking is strategic and often transactional; connections are built around projects, partnerships, and shared objectives. However, when I entered hospice and palliative care, I quickly realized that a supportive care network was something entirely different. In palliative care, building a network meant fostering genuine relationships across healthcare providers, community organizations, volunteers, and families to create an environment where patients' needs were met holistically.

One of my first realizations was that a robust network is essential for providing seamless care. When patients transition from hospitals to community care, or from home to hospice facilities, each handoff must be as smooth as possible. This requires not only logistical coordination but also emotional sensitivity and respect for each individual's unique journey. A well-established network helps ensure that patients and families experience continuity of care, no matter where they are in the journey.

Chapter 3: Building Connections – Establishing a Supportive Care Network

Lessons from the Front Lines: Learning through Experience

Early in my role, I was involved in establishing partnerships between tertiary and community hospitals, hospice organizations, and other healthcare providers. This experience highlighted the importance of aligning our goals and ensuring that everyone involved had a shared understanding of our mission. I recall several instances where patients were transferred to our care from hospital settings, often in fragile physical and emotional states. Each transition brought with it new challenges, from addressing unmet medical needs to helping families adjust to new care environments.

In the beginning, I approached these partnerships much as I would have in a corporate setting, with a focus on roles, responsibilities, and efficiency. However, I soon learned that collaboration in compassionate care required a different approach. Our partners needed to feel not only respected but also valued, understanding that they were integral to the care journey. Over time, I began to see that each person in our network, from social workers to volunteers, brought a unique perspective and expertise that enriched our overall mission. Embracing these relationships as genuine partnerships, rather than transactions, was key to building trust and establishing a care network that truly supported patients and families.

Leveraging Community Resources: Expanding the Circle of Care

One of the most impactful lessons I learned was the value of reaching out to local community resources. The Asia Pacific region is diverse, with vast differences in culture, language, and access to healthcare resources. By tapping into local community organizations, religious groups, and non-profit initiatives, we could extend our reach and provide culturally sensitive care that resonated with patients and families.

In serving and speaking with many volunteers and healthcare workers in low-resource settings, we observed the challenges of working in rural areas where access to healthcare is limited, and cultural beliefs about death and dying are deeply rooted in tradition. To outcome the barriers, one of the ways is to partner with a local community organization that provided education on palliative care to community leaders and elders, helping to bridge the gap between traditional beliefs and modern hospice practices. This partnership proved invaluable, as it helped us gain the trust of the community and paved the way for more open conversations about end-of-life care. Community organizations often have deep connections within their regions, making them essential allies in building a network of care that respects cultural norms and values.

Chapter 3: Building Connections – Establishing a Supportive Care Network

Building a Volunteer Network: The Heart of Hospice Care

Volunteers play an irreplaceable role in hospice and palliative care, offering companionship, emotional support, and practical assistance to patients and families. Building a network of committed volunteers was one of the most rewarding aspects of my work, and it taught me the importance of recognizing and nurturing the compassion that drives people to contribute their time and energy to this field.

One of my most memorable experiences was working with a group of volunteers who had come from various walks of life – retirees, young professionals, and even students eager to make a difference. Each volunteer brought a unique set of skills, whether it was listening, helping with daily tasks, or simply sitting with patients in silence. I quickly learned that our volunteers were the emotional backbone of our organization. Their dedication and selflessness added a layer of humanity that no clinical service could replicate.

Managing and supporting volunteers required a different approach than managing staff. Volunteers needed encouragement, a sense of purpose, and, most importantly, a community within the organization where they felt valued – regular training sessions, support groups, and debriefing meetings, creating a space where volunteers could share their experiences, learn from one another, and feel supported in their roles. Recognizing the personal impact of this work on volunteers was crucial to maintaining a sustainable volunteer network.

Creating Bridges Across Disciplines: Medical, Emotional, and Spiritual Support

In palliative care, addressing the whole person means bridging multiple disciplines — medical, emotional, spiritual, and social. Building a supportive care network required collaboration across these domains, ensuring that patients received comprehensive care that met their diverse needs.

A pivotal part of my learning process involved working with palliative care physicians, social workers, chaplains, and counsellors. Each discipline brought a unique perspective on how to support patients and families. For instance, I observed the impact that spiritual care providers could have on patients facing existential questions as they approached the end of life. One chaplain I worked with had an incredible ability to provide comfort to patients regardless of their religious beliefs, fostering peace and acceptance in a way that complemented the medical care they were receiving.

The support network extended beyond our walls, reaching out to home care providers, rehabilitation centres, and other facilities where patients might receive care at different stages of their journey. Establishing strong lines of communication with these external providers helped us coordinate care effectively and maintain continuity for our patients. Through regular check-ins, collaborative care plans, and shared goals, we were able to create a cohesive support network that prioritized the patient's needs above all else.

Chapter 3: Building Connections – Establishing a Supportive Care Network

Learning from Mentors and Colleagues: The Influence of Professor Cynthia Goh

Throughout my journey in hospice and palliative care, I was fortunate to work alongside Professor Cynthia Goh, a pioneer in the field who taught me invaluable lessons about the importance of a supportive care network. Professor Goh understood that palliative care could not thrive in isolation; it required collaboration, education, and a commitment to building connections across the healthcare continuum.

Professor Goh's approach to palliative care education was transformative. She believed that training healthcare providers in low-resource settings was not just about imparting knowledge; it was about creating a community of care that could support each other in the face of challenges. Working with her, I saw how she fostered connections between palliative care practitioners across Asia Pacific, bringing them together to share their experiences, learn from one another, and find solutions to common problems.

Professor Goh's dedication to building a collaborative network inspired me to approach my role with humility and openness. She taught me that the strength of a palliative care organization lies in its ability to connect with others, to learn continuously, and to adapt based on the needs of the community. Her influence remains a guiding force in my efforts to build a supportive care network that serves both patients and those who care for them.

Reflecting on the Impact of a Supportive Care Network

Looking back on my experiences, I realize that building a supportive care network is both an art and a science. It requires strategic planning, clear communication, and an unwavering commitment to compassion. My journey in hospice and palliative care has taught me that while corporate skills like resource management and operational efficiency are valuable, they must be applied with sensitivity and a focus on collaboration.

Each connection we build, whether with a hospital, community organization, or volunteer, adds to the strength of the network and enhances our ability to provide compassionate care. In a field where every interaction matters, building a network is not just about efficiency; it's about creating an environment where patients feel supported, families feel valued, and caregivers feel empowered.

A Network for the Future

As I work to build and strengthen this vision of a compassionate, sustainable network of care, my goal remains clear: to create a system that serves the needs of patients, families, and communities with resilience and compassion. Each relationship we cultivate, every partnership we foster, and each volunteer we support contributes to a future where hospice and palliative care are accessible, deeply compassionate, and enduring. This journey has shown me that building connections is one of the most meaningful ways we can

Chapter 3: Building Connections – Establishing a Supportive Care Network

serve — a network that stands as a testament to the power of compassion in action.

Today, I am still very much a learner. I'm fortunate to have access to a wealth of knowledge and guidance from Professor Cynthia Goh's legacy. Her remarkable network of beneficiaries — her peers, her students, her patients, and her contacts across the region — continues to be a rich source of learning and inspiration for me. After her passing, I've been deeply moved to see so many of her colleagues and students step forward to carry on her work, strengthening and expanding her vision for palliative and hospice care across the Asia Pacific region. The powerful network she established lives on, enabling me and many others to build upon her foundation of compassionate care.

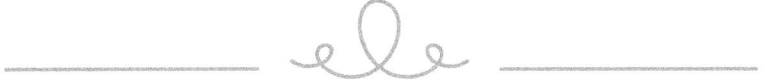

Chapter 4:
Financial Realities – Striving for Sustainability in Care

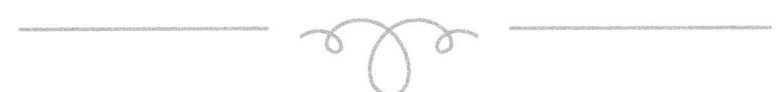

Entering the world of hospice and palliative care, I quickly recognized that the financial landscape here was vastly different from what I had experienced as Chief of Staff in a multinational firm. Managing a multi-million budget across global operations was no small feat, and in that role, I honed my skills in strategic planning, financial forecasting, and resource allocation. These experiences shaped my approach to managing resources, identifying priorities, and ensuring that every dollar served a purpose. But when it came to palliative care, I was an amateur – a newcomer with much to learn.

Yet, I knew there was a significant role for the financial skills I'd built over decades in corporate administration. Hospice and palliative care services are critically underfunded particularly in low-resource settings, and even in the high resource settings, the sustainability of these services is often a challenge. Balancing compassion with practicality became my mission, as I sought ways to adapt my corporate expertise to ensure a financially resilient and sustainable organization.

Understanding the Financial Realities in the Healthcare settings

In my corporate career, financial success was tied to maximizing returns, optimizing resource use, and ensuring that investments yielded measurable results. In hospice care, financial success meant something different – delivering the highest possible quality of care with often limited resources. Here, "return on investment" meant improving patient comfort, enhancing family support, and delivering care with dignity. It was a new perspective, one that took me out of the boardroom and into the world of patients and their families, whose needs were deeply human rather than financial.

When I took on a leadership role in a non-profit dedicated to healthcare, the reality of limited resources quickly set in. Unlike in the corporate world, where budgets could often be stretched to accommodate new initiatives, here every dollar was scrutinized, and every decision had to be made with sustainability in mind. This realization pushed me to think creatively about how to adapt corporate financial strategies to the unique demands of compassionate care.

Lesson One: Resource Optimization

In my previous role, resource optimization was a core part of my job. Managing a multi-million budget meant every line item was scrutinized for efficiency. I developed an instinct for identifying areas where resources could be reallocated or streamlined to maximize impact without compromising quality. This skill proved invaluable in the health care settings, where budgets are often tight, and every dollar needs to be stretched.

From my experience, one of the first areas I focused on was examining operational costs. Administrative expenses, while necessary, needed to be carefully controlled so that more of our funds could be directed toward patient care — implementing a lean approach, cutting down on unnecessary expenses, negotiating better rates with suppliers, and investing in technology that could streamline administrative tasks. By optimizing our operational budget, we were able to direct more resources toward clinical care, where it was most needed.

One significant example I have experienced involved a Ministry of Health initiative to create a seamless flow of patient care across acute hospitals, community hospitals, and home care. A single budget was allocated across these three settings, raising the complex question of how funds should be divided to best serve the patient. While we applied the Lean Six Sigma methodology to optimize costs scientifically, the true key to success was focusing on patient-centred care. We considered how each patient could transition smoothly from one care setting to another, prioritizing their well-being and preparing families for the care journey. By aligning patient information, care goals, and budgetary resources around the individual's needs, we optimized costs without compromising quality. In this way, compassionate care was achieved by integrating scientific methodology with a focus on the patient's best interests.

Staffing was another critical area where resource optimization became essential. In any healthcare setting, the largest expense is typically staffing, encompassing not only salaries but also training, benefits, and retention efforts. While maintaining a high standard of care was always a top priority, I quickly learned that we needed to be strategic about scheduling and task allocation to optimize resources effectively. By helping staff prioritize tasks and ensuring that roles were clearly defined, we were able to reduce overtime costs and improve overall efficiency. Every resource saved in this way went directly back into improving patient care.

To further enhance efficiency, we introduced flexible work hours, which allowed staff to better balance their shifts and personal lives while ensuring that patient needs were met around the clock. We also used Gantt charts to map out daily and weekly responsibilities, making it easier to allocate time precisely for each task and reduce overlap in responsibilities. This structured approach helped clarify individual duties, minimized inefficiencies, and allowed us to schedule staff more strategically. Additionally, we explored outsourcing administrative tasks such as billing, data entry, and scheduling to specialized providers. By shifting these non-clinical responsibilities outside the core team, we freed up clinical staff to focus solely on patient care. To supplement our resources, we brought in volunteers for non-medical tasks, such as companionship visits for patients and general support for families, which contributed significantly to patient comfort and care without straining our budget.

Partnering with corporate entities also proved beneficial. Many companies were willing to contribute resources or sponsor specific services as part of their corporate social responsibility initiatives. These partnerships allowed us to access additional support for specific needs, such as transportation services, equipment donations, or technology upgrades, which would otherwise have been financially challenging. We also adopted creative staffing solutions, such as job-sharing and cross-training, to make the best use of our existing team. Cross-training clinical and support staff allowed us to quickly adapt to fluctuating demands, ensuring that we always had team members available with the appropriate skills to handle varied patient needs.

These combined efforts proved that resource optimization is not only possible in a healthcare setting but also essential for providing sustainable, high-quality patient care. Through a combination of flexible scheduling, strategic outsourcing, corporate partnerships, and innovative staff utilization, we were able to maintain a compassionate, efficient, and resilient care environment that placed patient needs at the forefront.

Lesson Two: Revenue Diversification

One of the key principles I learned in corporate finance was the importance of revenue diversification. In the corporate world, relying on a single income stream was risky; diversifying our revenue sources helped buffer against fluctuations and provided stability. This principle applies even more critically in healthcare, where funding often depends on a narrow base of grants, donations, and government support.

Early on, I realized that relying solely on grants and donations was not a sustainable strategy for our organization. Grants are competitive, donations fluctuate, and government funding can be unpredictable. Drawing from my corporate experience, I began exploring ways to diversify our income sources. This included building partnerships with other organizations, developing private pay services, and looking for opportunities to collaborate with the private sector.

We introduced specialized workshops and training programs for healthcare providers, offering paid educational sessions on palliative care practices. This provided an additional revenue stream while also spreading knowledge about palliative care — a dual benefit that aligned with our mission. Additionally, we explored partnerships with corporate sponsors interested in supporting our cause, creating win-win opportunities where they could fulfil their social responsibility goals while we gained much-needed financial support.

Lesson Three: Building Financial Resilience through Strategic Planning

In corporate finance, strategic planning is essential for long-term success. As Chief of Staff responsible for annual financial budgeting, reporting, and control, I developed an approach to planning that balanced current needs with future growth. In healthcare, where resources are tight and demand is growing, strategic planning is even more critical.

To build financial resilience, one could begin implementing multi-year budgeting. While short-term budgets are necessary, multi-year budgeting helped us plan for growth and anticipate challenges in advance. This approach allowed us to allocate funds for long-term projects, such as training programs for local healthcare providers, that could strengthen our network over time.

An essential part of our strategic planning was establishing an emergency fund. In the corporate world, a cash reserve is critical for weathering unexpected downturns, and I quickly recognized the same need within a healthcare setting. With unpredictable funding sources, having a reserve fund meant we could continue operations during lean times and respond to unexpected challenges. Building this reserve required discipline and sacrifices, but the peace of mind and stability it provided was invaluable.

Though I am still learning, and my tenure in palliative and hospice care is relatively short, I have managed, step by step, to use these principles to strengthen the organization's financial foundation.

Through steady, incremental efforts — taking baby steps, really — we succeeded in increasing the organization's reserves fourfold over the years. This growth allowed us to expand the team's coverage and reach, providing greater support to those we serve.

Lesson Four: The Power of Financial Transparency and Accountability

In my corporate role, financial reporting and accountability were essential for maintaining the trust of shareholders and stakeholders. In hospice care, financial transparency was equally important for building trust with donors, staff, and the communities we served. Many of our donors wanted to know that their contributions were making a difference, and transparent financial reporting was one way to demonstrate our impact.

I introduced regular financial reports that outlined how funds were being used, focusing on the direct impact of donor contributions. For instance, rather than simply reporting on administrative expenses, we highlighted the percentage of funds usage. Every fundraising effort will be coupled its efficiency ratio and meeting all guidelines set by the Charity of Commissioner. This transparency not only built trust with our donors but also fostered a culture of accountability within the organization. Every member of our team understood that each dollar spent had to be justified by its impact on patient care.

It was a proud moment for all of us when, in the organization's 23rd year, we were awarded the Charity Transparency Award from the

Ministry. This recognition was a testament to the dedication and hard work of every level of the team. Together, we have demonstrated that a clear, mission-driven approach to resource management not only strengthens the organization but also brings tangible benefits to our community.

Lesson Five: Sustainable Growth through Collaboration and Innovation

In the corporate world, growth is driven by innovation and collaboration, and I found the same principle could apply in hospice care. While direct profits were not the goal, sustainable growth meant expanding our reach, improving our services, and ensuring long-term viability. I focused on building partnerships with local healthcare organizations, educational institutions, and community leaders. These partnerships helped us share resources, exchange knowledge, and collaborate on initiatives that could benefit the broader community.

For example, partnering with local universities allowed us to offer internships and training programs, which brought in additional support for our organization while providing invaluable experience for students interested in palliative care. These students often went on to become champions for palliative care in their own communities, extending our mission beyond our immediate reach.

Innovation was also crucial. In my corporate role, I had seen the benefits of investing in technology, and I applied the same mindset here. By investing in telehealth capabilities, for example, we could reach patients in remote areas, reducing transportation costs and improving access to care. This approach was not only cost-effective but also aligned with our mission to provide compassionate care to all, regardless of location.

The Challenge of Balancing Compassion with Financial Realism

One of the most challenging aspects of adapting corporate financial strategies to hospice care was balancing compassion with financial realism. In this field, every decision impacts lives directly, and cutting costs is never a simple matter. I found myself constantly evaluating how to maintain high-quality care while staying within budget.

This experience taught me that sustainability in hospice care requires both a heart for compassion and a mind for practicality. For example, while it was tempting to provide extensive services to every patient, I had to consider the long-term viability of our organization. This meant making difficult choices about prioritizing certain services based on need and impact. By involving the entire team in these decisions, we created a culture of shared responsibility, where everyone understood the importance of balancing care with sustainability.

Reflecting on My Journey: From Corporate to Compassionate Care

Looking back on my journey from corporate finance to hospice and palliative care, I am grateful for the skills I was able to bring with me and the lessons I've learned along the way. Striving for financial sustainability in compassionate care is not simply about numbers; it's about creating a framework that allows compassionate care to thrive despite financial limitations.

By merging corporate strategies with a commitment to patient-centered care, I hope to contribute to a future where hospice and palliative care organizations can continue to provide essential services to those in need. Every budget line, every resource allocation, and every partnership, is now motivated by a deeper purpose — a purpose rooted in compassion, dignity, and respect for the journey that every patient and family faces.

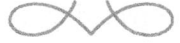

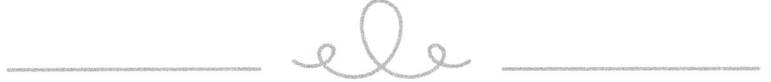

Chapter 5:
Leading with Empathy – Shifting from Corporate to Compassionate Leadership

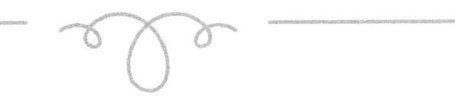

Transitioning from a corporate mindset to one rooted in compassion was a journey that required me to rethink what it meant to lead. In the corporate world, leadership often emphasizes performance, productivity, and efficiency – qualities that are critical in a business environment but needed recalibration in hospice and palliative care, where the priorities are more about supporting others through one of life's most profound journeys. The challenges of working in hospice care – witnessing the fragility of life and supporting families through loss – required a shift in leadership style that was as much about empathy and resilience as it was about structure and results.

In this new context, I came to understand the importance of leading with empathy, an approach deeply inspired by my father's teachings and his example as a devout Buddhist. My father taught me that leadership and compassion are intertwined, and that empathy is not only a skill but a way of being that defines how we interact with others, especially during difficult times. His teachings served as my guiding light, helping me build a supportive team and maintain morale in a field that inevitably confronts loss and grief.

Learning Compassion from My Father

My father was a faithful Buddhist who embodied the principles of compassion and mindfulness in everything he did. He taught me that true compassion goes beyond simply feeling sympathy; it requires a genuine commitment to alleviating the suffering of others. One lesson he often shared with me was rooted in the Buddhist principle of "Metta," or loving-kindness, which encourages us to approach every interaction with goodwill and a sincere desire for others to be well.

"Hatred does not cease by hatred, but only by love; this is the eternal rule," my father would say, quoting the Dhammapada, one of Buddhism's ancient texts. This teaching resonated with me, even more so after I transitioned into hospice care. My father's words taught me to approach others with an open heart, to see beyond their

Chapter 5: Leading with Empathy – Shifting from Corporate to Compassionate Leadership

exterior and understand their suffering and needs. In the corporate world, my focus had often been on achieving tangible goals and outcomes, but in hospice care, I realized that my role was to create a space of compassion and support for both my team and the patients and families we served.

One experience with my father particularly stands out. He once told me the story of how, during his own difficult times, he chose to respond with kindness to those who had wronged him. His calm and forgiving nature puzzled me, especially since I had often been taught that respect and recognition were things to be earned or demanded in the corporate world. But my father showed me that respect comes naturally when it is given freely and that love and kindness often yield the strongest influence.

This principle of loving-kindness became a foundation for how I approached leadership in role in palliative and hospice care. I learned that to be an effective leader, particularly in a field that deals with life's most delicate moments, I needed to lead with compassion, empathy, and a willingness to understand the emotional needs of my team.

The Challenges of Leading with Empathy

Shifting from a corporate leadership style to a compassionate, empathetic approach was not without its challenges. In my corporate career, I had been trained to make swift decisions, to prioritize efficiency, and to focus on measurable results. In hospice care, however, the emphasis was on patience, understanding, and emotional support — qualities that are not always easy to measure or quantify.

One of the first challenges I faced was learning to balance empathy with accountability. In hospice and palliative care, our work can be emotionally draining, and maintaining a high level of care requires both sensitivity and discipline. There were times when I struggled with how to address issues of performance or responsibility without undermining the compassionate environment we had worked to create. I learned that leading with empathy doesn't mean lowering expectations; it means recognizing the pressures that my team faces and supporting them in a way that empowers them to succeed.

For example, when a member of our team was going through personal difficulties, I found myself torn between the needs of the organization and my desire to support them. In a corporate setting, I might have prioritized the organization's goals and addressed performance issues more directly. But in this environment, I recognized the importance of being present and supportive, offering the time and space for them to navigate their personal challenges. By creating a compassionate atmosphere, I found that the team member was not only able to overcome their difficulties but returned with renewed dedication and appreciation for the support they had received.

Chapter 5: Leading with Empathy – Shifting from Corporate to Compassionate Leadership

Building a Supportive Team in a Challenging Field

One of the greatest rewards of leading with empathy in hospice and palliative care has been building a supportive and resilient team. Working in a field where we are constantly faced with loss requires an environment where team members feel valued, supported, and connected to one another. To foster this sense of community, I began implementing practices that encouraged open communication, emotional support, and professional growth.

I introduced regular team meetings where we could discuss not only operational matters but also our emotional experiences. These meetings became a safe space for sharing the challenges of our work, the joy of helping others, and the grief that sometimes accompanied it. I noticed that as we opened up to one another, the team grew closer and more supportive. They felt less isolated in their experiences and more connected to our shared mission. In these moments, I could see how leading with empathy was not only beneficial to individual team members but also strengthened the overall resilience of our organization.

One valuable lesson I learned was the importance of acknowledging the emotional labour involved in hospice care. I encouraged team members to take time for self-care, to lean on each other, and to seek support when they needed it. This focus on well-being became a central part of our organization's culture, helping us maintain morale and prevent burnout in a field that is emotionally demanding. By placing empathy at the core of our leadership approach, we were able to build a team that was not only skilled but deeply committed to our mission.

Maintaining Morale in a Field Often Touched by Loss

Working in any healthcare settings, especially hospice care, means facing the reality of loss on a daily basis. For our team, this is both a privilege and a challenge. Witnessing the resilience and grace of patients and their families is inspiring, but it also requires us to confront our own emotions and vulnerabilities. Leading with empathy has taught me that maintaining morale in this environment requires a balance of compassion, resilience, and gratitude.

One practice I implemented was regular reflection sessions, where we would take time to recognize the impact of our work. These sessions allowed us to celebrate small victories, such as a patient's comfort during their final days or a family's gratitude for the support they received. Reflecting on these moments helped remind the team of the profound importance of their work, even amid the sadness that often accompanies it. I realized that gratitude and appreciation are powerful tools for maintaining morale and reinforcing the purpose that drives us.

Another important aspect of maintaining morale was ensuring that our team had access to resources for emotional support. I worked to establish partnerships with counsellors and mental health professionals who could provide support to team members as needed. Just as we care for our patients, I saw it as my responsibility to care for the emotional well-being of my team. By creating an environment where team members felt supported, valued, and understood, we were able to foster resilience and continue our work with compassion.

The Rewards of Leading with Empathy

Although the transition from corporate to compassionate leadership was challenging, the rewards have been immense. Leading with empathy has allowed me to build a team that is not only effective but deeply connected to our mission. Each team member brings their whole self to their work, knowing that they are valued for who they are and supported in what they do. This sense of purpose and connection has made our organization stronger, more resilient, and better equipped to provide the highest quality of care to our patients and families.

In the end, my father's teachings on compassion and loving-kindness have become the foundation of my leadership philosophy. His lesson that "hatred does not cease by hatred, but only by love" has guided me through difficult decisions, reminded me of the power of empathy, and inspired me to lead with a compassionate heart. As I continue on this journey, I am grateful for the opportunity to bring my corporate skills into this field in a way that honours my father's wisdom and embodies the principles of compassionate care.

Leading with empathy has transformed not only my approach to leadership but also my understanding of what it means to serve. In hospice care, our work goes beyond tasks and outcomes; it is about creating an environment where patients, families, and team members feel seen, supported, and valued. This journey has taught me that true leadership is not about authority or control; it is about compassion, understanding, and the commitment to make a difference in the lives of others.

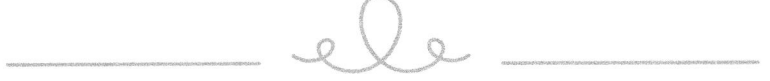

Chapter 6:
Embracing Technology – Modern Tools for Patient-Centered Care

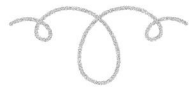

In recent years, the role of technology in healthcare has expanded dramatically, bringing both opportunities and challenges. Nowhere is this more evident than in hospice and palliative care, where the delicate balance between technology and compassion must be carefully managed. Reflecting on my corporate background, I can see the vast potential that technology holds for enhancing patient care, from telehealth to advanced data management. However, in hospice care, technology must serve the human connection rather than replace it.

One of the most profound lessons on the importance of technology in patient care came not from my corporate experience but from a deeply personal one: the time my mother was hospitalized in the ICU during the pandemic. Her stay in the ICU underscored the ways technology can bridge distances, provide comfort, and support patient-centred care when in-person connection is limited. My mother's fighting spirit and resilience became my inspiration, and her experience opened my eyes to the profound role technology can play in palliative care without sacrificing the human touch.

The Pandemic: A Turning Point for Technology in Care

The COVID-19 pandemic disrupted every aspect of healthcare, and hospice and palliative care were no exception. As hospitals and care facilities restricted visitation to prevent the spread of the virus, families were left disconnected from their loved ones, often during the most critical moments. My mother was one of those patients, placed in an ICU with limited visitation. It was a painful experience, one that left our family feeling helpless as we longed to be by her side.

However, technology provided a bridge in ways I had never anticipated. Through video calls and virtual meetings facilitated by the hospital, we were able to see her face, talk to her, and offer her encouragement, albeit from a distance. This experience showed me firsthand the role technology can play in maintaining family connections, especially in hospice and palliative care where the presence of loved ones is so vital. While I had always seen technology as a tool for efficiency and data management in my corporate life, I came to realize its power to foster emotional connection and support in healthcare.

My mother's strength and resilience through her illness inspired me to continue exploring how technology could be integrated into hospice care without losing the essential human touch. In many ways, it felt as though she was teaching me a lesson on the importance of compassionate care, even as she fought her own battle. This experience reshaped my understanding of technology's role in palliative care and motivated me to explore how modern tools can enhance patient-centred care.

Telehealth: Bridging Distance and Expanding Access to Care

Telehealth has emerged as a powerful tool in hospice and palliative care, allowing healthcare providers to reach patients who might otherwise have limited access to services. In my mother's case, telehealth allowed us to remain present and connected to her, even when physical visits were restricted. This experience reinforced my belief that telehealth can play a vital role in maintaining family connections, as well as providing direct care to patients in their own homes.

In hospice and palliative care, telehealth enables providers to conduct virtual visits, monitor symptoms, and offer support to families remotely. This has been especially beneficial in rural or underserved areas, where access to specialized palliative care is often limited. Telehealth has the potential to reduce travel time, lower costs, and minimize the physical demands on patients who may be frail or in pain. By embracing telehealth, hospice organizations can ensure that patients and families receive the support they need, even if they are unable to visit a facility in person.

One of the key challenges I've encountered is balancing the benefits of telehealth with the need for personal, hands-on care. While telehealth can provide a level of comfort and support, it cannot replace the physical presence of a caregiver or the warmth of a human touch. In palliative care, where emotional and spiritual needs are as important as medical ones, telehealth must be used as a complement rather than a substitute. My experience with my mother in the ICU reminded me of this balance, as we cherished the video calls but still longed to be physically present with her. This taught me that technology can support, but never replace, the fundamental human elements of hospice care.

Data Management and Predictive Analytics: Enhancing Care Delivery

In my corporate role, data management and analytics were essential for making informed decisions, optimizing resources, and forecasting future needs. When I transitioned into hospice care, I saw the potential for these tools to enhance care delivery, especially in a field where understanding patient needs is critical.

Predictive analytics, for example, can help hospice providers identify patients who may benefit from early palliative care interventions. By analysing patient data, healthcare teams can anticipate symptoms, adjust care plans, and allocate resources more effectively. For example, predictive models can help identify patients at higher risk of pain crises or hospitalizations, allowing providers to intervene proactively and improve patient comfort.

In my mother's case, we were grateful for the continuous monitoring systems in place in the ICU, which allowed her healthcare team to detect changes in her condition in real-time. This gave us peace of mind, knowing that her care team was aware of her needs and could respond quickly. In hospice care, predictive analytics can offer a similar level of support by enabling providers to anticipate needs, personalize care, and provide patients and families with a sense of security.

However, integrating data analytics into hospice care requires a thoughtful approach to protect patient privacy and maintain the personal, individualized nature of care. Data management tools must be used to enhance, not overshadow, the compassionate interactions that are at the heart of hospice work. By using data to inform decisions, providers can create a more responsive and supportive care environment while honouring the unique needs of each patient.

Digital Health Records: Streamlining Communication and Improving Continuity of Care

Digital health records have transformed the way patient information is managed, allowing healthcare providers to share information more easily and ensure continuity of care. In hospice and palliative care, where patients may move between different care settings — home, hospital, and hospice — having a centralized digital health record can be invaluable.

Reflecting on my corporate experience, I recognized the value of efficient information flow and clear communication. In hospice care, a digital health record enables providers to keep track of patient preferences, symptoms, and treatment plans, allowing for seamless transitions between caregivers. This continuity is particularly important in end-of-life care, where changes in providers or settings can be disorienting for patients and families.

When my mother was in the ICU, the healthcare team's ability to access her records instantly made her care more coordinated and efficient. There were fewer delays in treatment, less confusion about her medical history, and greater confidence on our part that her care team was fully informed. In hospice care, a similar approach can improve the patient experience, reduce errors, and ensure that every provider involved in a patient's care has access to the information they need.

Virtual Support Groups: Offering Comfort and Community to Families

Hospice care often extends beyond the patient to include emotional support for family members. In my mother's case, being able to connect virtually with other family members who were also concerned about her well-being provided us with comfort and solidarity. Inspired by this, I recognized the potential of virtual support groups in hospice care, where family members may need additional support as they navigate the emotional challenges of losing a loved one.

Virtual support groups allow families to connect with others who understand their experience, share their feelings, and receive guidance from trained facilitators. This can be especially beneficial for family members who live far away or who are unable to attend in-person meetings. By providing virtual support options, hospice organizations can offer families a sense of community and reduce feelings of isolation.

These support groups serve as a reminder that technology can foster connection and compassion, even when in-person interactions are not possible. In the case of my mother's illness, these virtual gatherings gave our family a sense of unity and hope. In hospice care, virtual support groups can offer a similar lifeline to families facing the loss of a loved one.

Balancing Technology with Human-Centered Care

Reflecting on my journey, I have come to realize that the integration of technology in hospice care requires a careful balance. Technology should serve as a bridge, not a barrier, to human connection. It must be implemented in ways that support compassionate care, not replace it. My experience with my mother's illness taught me that while technology can provide comfort and convenience, it is the human connection — whether through a voice on a video call, a compassionate message, or a shared moment — that truly makes a difference.

In hospice and palliative care, technology can enhance patient-centred care by increasing access, improving communication, and enabling proactive interventions. However, we must remain mindful of the need to preserve the essence of palliative care, which is rooted in empathy, respect, and dignity. Technology is a tool that can support our work, but it must never overshadow the human touch that is essential in this field.

Moving Forward with Compassionate Technology

As I continue my journey in hospice care, I am committed to embracing technology in ways that align with our mission of compassionate, patient-centred care. My mother's fighting spirit during her time in the ICU serves as a reminder that every interaction, whether digital or in person, has the potential to provide comfort and strength. Her resilience taught me that technology can be a

Chapter 6: Embracing Technology – Modern Tools for Patient-Centered Care

powerful ally in palliative care, but only when it is used thoughtfully and with a focus on the patient's experience.

In the end, technology should serve as a means to enhance the compassionate work we do, allowing us to extend our reach and support patients and families in meaningful ways. As we navigate this evolving landscape, I am often reminded of the lessons I learned during my mother's illness – lessons that have guided my approach to integrating technology in compassionate care. Her journey continues to inspire me, reinforcing the importance of balancing innovation with empathy, so that we may offer the best possible care to those who need it most.

While my mother has passed on, technology has continued to progress, new illnesses emerge, and patients face increasingly complex health challenges. One of the breakthroughs of today is the advancement of artificial intelligence. I often wonder how AI might have made a difference during my mother's last days. Could AI have provided more seamless ways to connect patients with their family members? Might it have helped to ensure that she lived her remaining days with dignity and freedom from pain?

As I ponder the future, I am hopeful that AI and other emerging technologies will open new possibilities in hospice and palliative care. These tools may help bridge the gap between patients and their loved ones, improving communication and comfort during the most vulnerable times. It's a humbling thought that the work we do today, together with future innovations, could help bring relief, connection, and compassion to those who need it most.

A New Path: My Journey from Corporate into Hospice and Palliative Care Leadership

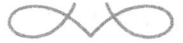

Chapter 7: Community Engagement – The Power of Building Trust

One of the essential aspects of hospice and palliative care is its connection to the community. Unlike other areas of healthcare, where patients may be isolated within the hospital environment, hospice care extends to homes, families, and the broader community. As I transitioned from corporate administration to the world of hospice care, I came to understand that community support is not just beneficial – it is vital. Hospice organizations thrive on the trust and engagement of the communities they serve. Without it, we would struggle to reach patients, educate families, and advocate for compassionate end-of-life care.

In my corporate life, community engagement was often driven by brand-building, market outreach, and partnerships that aimed to generate financial returns. In hospice care, community engagement is about building relationships, fostering trust, and ensuring that the values of dignity and compassion are at the forefront. This chapter explores the strategies I've observed and the lessons I've learned from others in building trust within the community to support hospice care, drawing parallels with corporate strategies and adapting them for a purpose-driven mission.

Observing the Importance of Community Trust in Hospice Care

Early on in my hospice journey, I witnessed the profound impact that community trust can have on a hospice organization. Patients and families often feel vulnerable when faced with end-of-life decisions, and their willingness to embrace hospice care relies heavily on their trust in the organization and its mission. Unlike in a corporate setting, where trust can be built through consistent brand messaging and customer service, trust in hospice care requires a deeper, more personal connection. It is about showing families that their loved ones will be treated with dignity, that their emotional and spiritual needs will be honoured, and that they will be supported through the grieving process.

One example that stood out to me was an outreach program I observed at a hospice organization serving a culturally diverse community. This organization recognized that different cultural backgrounds had unique perspectives on death and dying, and it tailored its approach to meet the specific needs of each group. Staff members held informational sessions in community centres, places of worship, and local organizations where they could connect with people in familiar and trusted environments. By showing respect for cultural differences and engaging with communities on their own terms, the organization built a strong foundation of trust. It was a lesson for me in the power of respect and cultural sensitivity in building community relationships.

Learning to Adapt Corporate Outreach Strategies to a Community Mission

In my corporate career, I learned the importance of outreach strategies to build brand loyalty and awareness. These strategies typically involved targeted messaging, strategic partnerships, and a clear value proposition. In hospice care, I realized that these principles could be adapted to serve a mission-driven purpose. However, the language, goals, and methods needed to be transformed to align with the values of compassion, empathy, and respect for patient dignity.

For example, I observed that successful hospice organizations applied outreach strategies similar to those used in corporate public relations. They used clear, empathetic messaging to educate the community about hospice care, debunking misconceptions and explaining the benefits of palliative care services. Through workshops, public talks, and collaboration with local media, they created awareness that was both informative and reassuring. These efforts were not aimed at "selling" hospice care but at building understanding and trust within the community.

I also saw the importance of transparency and open communication in outreach efforts. Families want to know that their loved ones will be well cared for, and communities want to understand how hospice organizations operate. Some hospice organizations held annual open days, inviting community members to tour the facility, meet the staff, and ask questions. This transparency helped demystify hospice care, creating a sense of openness and accessibility that fostered trust and encouraged more people to consider hospice services for their loved ones.

Building Partnerships with Local Organizations and Religious Institutions

In the corporate world, partnerships with other organizations often serve to expand reach, tap into new markets, or strengthen a brand's image. In hospice care, partnerships have the added purpose of supporting patients' emotional and spiritual needs, which are just as important as their physical care. During my time in hospice care, I observed how partnerships with local organizations, religious institutions, and community groups strengthened the trust between hospice providers and the communities they served.

For example, in one hospice organization I observed, partnerships were built with local religious institutions to provide spiritual support to patients and families. Recognizing that faith is a source of comfort for many, the hospice organization reached out to various religious leaders who could provide counselling, prayers, and support that aligned with the spiritual needs of different faiths. This partnership not only enriched the care experience but also helped the community see the hospice as a place that respected and supported their beliefs and values.

These partnerships also extended to local charities and support groups, such as grief counselling organizations and volunteer groups. By working together, these organizations created a network of support for families, offering resources that the hospice itself might not have been able to provide alone. I learned that by fostering these connections, hospice organizations could multiply their impact, expanding their reach and enriching the support available to patients and families.

Emphasizing Education and Awareness

One of the most significant barriers to hospice care is a lack of understanding or misconceptions about what hospice entails. In corporate settings, educating the market about a product or service is often the first step in building acceptance. In hospice care, education serves a similar function but with a deeper purpose. People need to understand that hospice care is about quality of life, not simply end-of-life, and that it provides essential support to both patients and families.

I've observed organizations that emphasize community education through seminars, informational workshops, and partnerships with healthcare providers. For instance, some hospice umbrella bodies offer free seminars to educate the public about the benefits of early palliative care, symptom management, and support services for families. This approach, which I recognized as akin to corporate educational outreach, proved invaluable in raising awareness and reducing the stigma associated with hospice care.

In one powerful example, a hospice organization partnered with a local hospital to provide training sessions for primary care doctors, nurses, and social workers on how to discuss hospice care with patients and families. By educating healthcare professionals, the hospice organization extended its outreach indirectly, as these professionals could then educate their patients and encourage them to consider hospice services. This approach was a testament to how education could serve as a bridge, connecting hospice care providers with the broader healthcare community and fostering trust along the way.

Engaging Volunteers: A Pillar of Community Trust

Volunteers play a vital role in hospice care, providing companionship to patients, supporting families, and assisting with day-to-day tasks. In corporate settings, volunteerism often aligns with corporate social responsibility, fostering goodwill and brand loyalty. In hospice care, however, volunteers embody the spirit of compassion and selflessness, reinforcing the trust and connection between the organization and the community.

During my journey in the healthcare settings, I learned that recruiting and training volunteers requires a deep commitment to building a supportive, inclusive environment. Volunteers often come from the community itself, and their presence within the hospice is a powerful testament to the community's belief in and support for the organization. I observed hospices that had created rigorous training programs to ensure that volunteers were well-prepared, both practically and emotionally, for the challenges of hospice work. By providing comprehensive training, these hospices showed respect for the volunteers' roles, reinforcing the sense of trust within the organization and the community.

In one memorable instance, a hospice organization held an annual volunteer recognition event, inviting the community to celebrate the contributions of its volunteers. This event not only honored the volunteers but also allowed community members to see firsthand the commitment and compassion that define hospice care. The celebration strengthened the bond between the hospice and the community, as volunteers shared their stories and experiences, giving the community a more personal, relatable perspective on the work being done.

Observing the Impact of Transparency and Accountability

In corporate settings, transparency and accountability are often used to build investor confidence and customer loyalty. In hospice care, these principles serve to build trust with the community. Families want to know how their donations are used, and the community wants assurance that the hospice organization is acting ethically and responsibly.

I observed several hospice organizations that practiced transparency by regularly publishing reports, hosting open meetings, and sharing success stories. They provided details on how funds were allocated, how many patients they served, and what future initiatives were planned. This openness helped community members see the direct impact of their support and provided assurance that their donations were being used wisely.

In one case, a hospice organization published an annual report that included patient testimonials, family stories, and data on patient outcomes. This report served as both a transparency tool and a powerful way to engage the community. By sharing the personal impact of their work, the hospice organization reinforced the community's trust and encouraged further support.

Building a Legacy of Trust through Compassionate Care

Throughout my journey, I've come to understand that community engagement in hospice care is not just about outreach, partnerships, or volunteerism; it's about building a legacy of trust. Community support is a testament to the values that hospice organizations stand for: compassion, dignity, and respect for the individual. Each partnership, each educational effort, and each act of transparency contributes to a foundation of trust that supports the organization and allows it to serve with integrity.

In hospice care, trust is not something that can be bought or branded; it is earned through consistent, compassionate actions that demonstrate a commitment to the community. The lessons I've observed and the strategies I've learned along the way have shown me that community engagement is not merely a strategic initiative but a responsibility that lies at the heart of hospice care. Building trust within the community empowers hospice organizations to fulfil their mission, support patients and families, and continue the compassionate work that defines hospice and palliative care.

As I continue my work, I am reminded that the support of the community is a powerful force, one that sustains us through challenges and inspires us to keep serving. It is a privilege to build and nurture these relationships, knowing that together, we can create a supportive, compassionate environment for those in need.

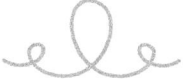

Chapter 8:
Navigating Compliance – Balancing Mission with Regulatory Demands

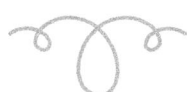

Navigating the legal and regulatory landscape in hospice and palliative care has been one of the most challenging aspects of my work in this field. Coming from a corporate background, I was accustomed to dealing with regulations and compliance requirements, but the complexities I encountered in hospice and palliative care were of an entirely different nature. This chapter delves into the unique regulatory and legal challenges in palliative care, particularly in regions where this form of care is not fully recognized as a medical specialty. From medication availability issues to cultural barriers and limited government strategies, the obstacles are numerous and often deeply entrenched.

Balancing these regulatory demands with our mission to deliver compassionate, patient-centred care has been a significant learning curve. Along the way, I've encountered challenges in understanding country-specific compliance requirements and witnessed the unique limitations faced by healthcare providers in low-resource settings. My journey into palliative care compliance has revealed just how critical advocacy, education, and strategic partnerships are in bringing compassionate care to those who need it most.

The Challenge of Palliative Care as an Unrecognized Specialty

One of the most foundational challenges we face is the fact that palliative care is not formally recognized as a medical specialty in many parts of the Asia Pacific region. Unlike oncology or cardiology, palliative care lacks a structured certification path, professional standards, and official recognition in some countries. This lack of recognition creates numerous compliance hurdles. Without an official specialty status, healthcare providers and organizations often struggle to secure funding, attract qualified staff, and implement standardized training programs.

In some countries, the absence of formal palliative care programs means there is little to no national framework or strategy to guide the development of hospice services. I recall learning about a neighbouring country where palliative care was limited to a few urban hospitals, with minimal availability in rural areas. Without government support or regulatory frameworks, organizations are left to navigate compliance on their own, often relying on improvised policies and volunteer training.

The lack of formal recognition also complicates our ability to communicate the value of palliative care to policymakers and healthcare institutions. I observed that when approaching healthcare administrators or government officials, the absence of an official palliative care specialty left us with few data-driven arguments or benchmarks to make our case. This made it difficult to advocate for increased support, resources, or regulatory adjustments to accommodate the needs of palliative care patients.

Medication Availability and Regulatory Barriers

Access to essential medications, particularly opioids for pain management, is another significant regulatory challenge in palliative care. Pain relief is a fundamental aspect of palliative care, yet stringent regulations on opioid distribution, along with bureaucratic hurdles, limit the availability of these medications in many countries. Regulations on opioid distribution, aimed at controlling misuse, inadvertently restrict legitimate access for patients who are suffering.

In some of the countries I've worked in, opioids are heavily regulated and only accessible through a limited number of healthcare facilities, often located in urban centres. For patients in rural areas, this means that access to effective pain relief is not just challenging — it is practically non-existent. Without access to these essential medications, patients endure unnecessary suffering, undermining the very purpose of palliative care.

One particularly striking example I encountered was in a rural area where morphine, the most commonly used opioid in palliative care, was unavailable. The lack of regulatory support for pain management created an enormous burden for healthcare providers and families alike. To mitigate these issues, I observed healthcare organizations working closely with government health ministries to advocate for regulatory changes that would allow for easier access to pain relief medication. These partnerships were often slow and bureaucratic, but they underscored the importance of persistence and advocacy in improving regulatory support for palliative care.

Cultural Barriers and Traditional Medicine

Another challenge I observed was the reliance on traditional medicine, especially in rural and underserved communities. In countries where palliative care services are limited or difficult to access, many patients turn to traditional healing methods as their primary means of care. This approach is often influenced by cultural beliefs, the lack of infrastructure, and the high cost of modern medical care. For families in rural areas, traditional medicine provides a form of comfort and connection to their heritage, especially when conventional healthcare seems out of reach.

For example, in one country I worked in, families from remote villages would often resort to herbal remedies and spiritual healers for end-of-life care. This practice was not necessarily due to a lack of trust in modern medicine but rather a result of limited access and affordability. Many of these families faced logistical and financial barriers to accessing formal healthcare, making natural healing methods and traditional medicine the only viable options.

Observing these cultural dynamics taught me the importance of respect and understanding. Rather than attempting to replace traditional practices, effective palliative care organizations sought to integrate these cultural elements into their care strategies. I observed healthcare providers working with traditional healers, collaborating to offer a blended approach that honoured cultural beliefs while providing modern symptom management. This approach not only respected the patient's background but also helped build trust within the community, encouraging more families to consider palliative care as an option.

The Financial Burden and Limited Understanding of Medical Costs

Another factor that complicates the compliance landscape is the financial burden associated with hospice care. The cost of modern healthcare is prohibitive for many families, particularly those in rural and low-income areas. I learned that for many people, the expense of palliative care — especially when compounded by the cost of medications, hospital visits, and travel — leads families to give up on seeking formal care altogether. Instead, they often rely on traditional healing or accept illness as a matter of fate and divine will.

This financial barrier is compounded by a general lack of understanding about the nature and purpose of palliative care. In some cases, families associate healthcare solely with curative treatments, and when faced with a terminal diagnosis, they may see no value in seeking additional care. This misconception presents a significant barrier to compliance, as healthcare providers struggle to communicate the importance of pain management, emotional support, and end-of-life care.

I recall an instance where a family in a rural area expressed confusion over the concept of palliative care. To them, healthcare was synonymous with treatment aimed at curing illness. When healthcare providers explained the role of palliative care in managing symptoms and improving quality of life, the family initially hesitated. Their reluctance reflected not only a lack of awareness but also the financial burden associated with extended care. This experience taught me the importance of community education in bridging the gap between medical costs and the value of hospice care, allowing families to make informed decisions about their loved ones' care.

Adapting Compliance Strategies to Local Contexts

One of the most valuable lessons I've learned in navigating compliance is the importance of adapting strategies to fit local contexts. In the corporate world, compliance often follows a one-size-

Chapter 8: Navigating Compliance – Balancing Mission with Regulatory Demands

fits-all approach driven by global standards. However, in palliative care, particularly in low-resource settings, compliance strategies must be flexible, culturally sensitive, and locally relevant.

I observed that successful hospice organizations adapted their compliance strategies by forming partnerships with local government agencies, healthcare providers, and community leaders. By working within existing structures, these organizations were able to navigate regulatory barriers more effectively. For instance, in one country where opioid regulations were strict, the hospice organization partnered with the health ministry to establish a pilot program that provided controlled access to pain relief medications. This collaborative approach allowed the organization to meet regulatory requirements while advocating for patients' needs.

Another key strategy I learned from observing others was the importance of incremental change. Regulatory barriers cannot always be dismantled overnight, but through small, consistent efforts, organizations can make progress. I saw examples of healthcare providers using case studies, patient testimonials, and data to gradually build support for palliative care within regulatory bodies. These incremental changes helped pave the way for broader policy adjustments, reflecting a commitment to both compliance and patient-centred care.

Advocacy and Education: A Path to Regulatory Progress

Perhaps the most important insight I gained from navigating compliance in hospice care is the power of advocacy and education. Compliance challenges often stem from a lack of understanding or awareness among policymakers, healthcare providers, and the public. By educating these stakeholders about the purpose and benefits of palliative care, organizations can foster greater acceptance and support for regulatory changes.

I observed that successful hospice organizations invested time and resources in advocacy campaigns, working to educate government officials, healthcare providers, and community leaders about the value of palliative care. By presenting data, sharing patient stories, and highlighting the need for compassionate care, these organizations-built momentum for regulatory reform. One organization hosted workshops and seminars, inviting policymakers to learn more about the benefits of palliative care and the specific regulatory adjustments needed to support its growth.

These advocacy efforts were instrumental in driving regulatory change. Through education, hospice organizations could bridge the gap between their mission and the requirements of compliance, gradually gaining the support needed to improve access to palliative care. Observing this taught me that compliance is not just about meeting existing standards but about advocating for change and educating stakeholders to support a compassionate approach to care.

Chapter 8: Navigating Compliance – Balancing Mission with Regulatory Demands

Balancing Mission with Compliance

Navigating compliance in hospice and palliative care requires a delicate balance between upholding regulatory requirements and staying true to the mission of compassionate care. In this field, regulations are not always designed with palliative care in mind, and they often reflect gaps in awareness, cultural differences, and resource limitations. Balancing these demands with the commitment to alleviate suffering, honour cultural beliefs, and support families through end-of-life care is a challenge that requires patience, advocacy, and adaptability.

My journey through the regulatory landscape has shown me that compliance in hospice care is as much about building relationships and fostering understanding as it is about following rules. By working with policymakers, educating communities, and respecting cultural values, we can navigate these challenges while staying true to the core mission of hospice and palliative care: to provide compassionate, patient-centred support that respects the dignity of every individual.

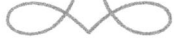

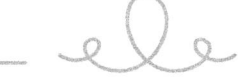

Chapter 9:
Measuring What Matters – Assessing Impact in a Care Network

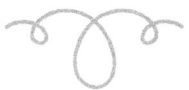

In hospice and palliative care, success cannot be measured solely by conventional metrics like revenue or growth. Unlike the corporate world, where performance indicators often focus on productivity and financial returns, hospice care requires a different approach to assessing impact. Here, what truly matters is the quality of care provided, patient satisfaction, and the organization's ability to fulfil its mission of compassionate end-of-life support.

Drawing on my corporate experience with performance metrics, I came to realize that assessing impact in hospice care requires a blend of traditional and mission-driven metrics. This chapter explores the ways we can measure success in hospice care, the challenges inherent in assessing intangible outcomes, and the critical role of frameworks like the Quality of Death Index in helping countries evaluate and improve their palliative care systems.

The Importance of Measuring What Matters

In the corporate world, metrics are used to gauge success and guide decision-making, ensuring that goals align with the organization's strategy. In hospice care, measuring impact serves a similar purpose but with a much more human-centred focus. Instead of simply tracking numbers, our metrics must capture the essence of compassionate care, quality of life, and the holistic well-being of patients and their families.

I learned early on that if we are to improve, grow, and advocate for hospice care, we must have data that demonstrates our impact. While the mission of providing dignified, compassionate end-of-life care may seem difficult to quantify, meaningful metrics allow us to assess our performance, identify areas for improvement, and communicate the value of our work to donors, policymakers, and the communities we serve. Metrics grounded in patient experience and quality of care help ensure that we remain focused on what truly matters: providing the highest possible standard of support to those at the end of life.

Chapter 9: Measuring What Matters – Assessing Impact in a Care Network

Core Metrics in Hospice Care

Drawing from my corporate background, I recognized that some of the principles used in business — such as measuring customer satisfaction, operational efficiency, and quality — could be adapted to hospice care to gauge performance effectively. The key was to identify metrics that aligned with our mission and goals. Here are some of the core metrics that have proven valuable in assessing impact within hospice care:

1. Quality of Care

Quality of care is the cornerstone of hospice work, encompassing the physical, emotional, and spiritual support provided to patients and their families. To measure quality, many hospice organizations use standardized assessments that track symptom management, patient comfort, and satisfaction with care. Quality indicators might include pain control, emotional support, and timely access to services. Patient and family feedback, gathered through surveys and follow-up interviews, helps us understand how well we are meeting the unique needs of each individual.

2. Patient and Family Satisfaction

Just as customer satisfaction is crucial in the corporate world, patient and family satisfaction is essential in hospice care. A high satisfaction rate indicates that families feel supported and that the care team is effectively meeting their needs. Surveys measuring satisfaction can include questions on the adequacy of communication, responsiveness of staff, and the overall experience. In hospice care, patient and family feedback offers invaluable insights into areas where we can improve and ensure that our approach remains patient-centred.

3. Operational Efficiency

Hospice care, like any other organization, must operate efficiently to maximize resources and provide sustainable services. Operational metrics, such as bed occupancy rates, time from referral to admission, and staff-to-patient ratios, provide insight into how effectively resources are being utilized. In the corporate world, efficiency often translates to cost savings; in hospice care, it means the ability to serve more patients and expand access to care. Effective resource allocation ensures that the organization can deliver high-quality care even within budget constraints.

4. Care Accessibility

Measuring access to hospice services is critical, especially in regions where palliative care is limited. Accessibility metrics can include the number of patients served in rural areas, availability of home-based services, and partnerships with local healthcare providers. By assessing accessibility, we ensure that we are reaching underserved populations and fulfilling our mission to provide equitable care to all who need it.

5. Staff Well-being and Retention

Staff well-being is an often-overlooked metric, but it is essential in hospice care, where the emotional demands of the job can lead to burnout. Measuring staff satisfaction and retention rates helps us understand the work environment and the support needs of our team. High staff turnover can disrupt continuity of care and affect the quality of patient interactions. Focusing on staff well-being enables us to foster a supportive workplace that, in turn, enhances patient care.

Learning from the Quality of Death Index

An important benchmark in the field of palliative care is the Quality of Death Index, that is commissioned by the Lien Foundation of Singapore, first published by The Economist Intelligence Unit in 2010 and updated in 2015. This index ranks countries on the quality of palliative care available, based on factors such as availability of pain relief, government involvement, public awareness, and overall quality of care. The Quality of Death Index has proven invaluable in helping countries understand their strengths and weaknesses in end-of-life care, serving as both a call to action and a framework for improvement.

For example, the 2015 Quality of Death Index revealed significant disparities in palliative care availability across countries, particularly between high-income and low-income nations. By highlighting these differences, the index brought global attention to the need for more equitable access to palliative care and provided policymakers with a roadmap for improvement. In some countries, the index prompted governments to develop national palliative care strategies, increase funding for hospice services, and improve access to pain relief medications.

From my perspective, the Quality of Death Index is a powerful reminder that data-driven insights can be transformative. When countries have access to reliable metrics, they are better equipped to make informed decisions, allocate resources effectively, and implement policies that enhance the quality of palliative care. Observing how this index has influenced policy changes in various regions taught me the importance of using metrics to advocate for improvements, not only within organizations but across entire healthcare systems.

Balancing Metrics with Compassionate Care

While metrics are invaluable in assessing impact, there is an inherent risk in becoming overly focused on numbers. In the corporate world, performance metrics often drive decisions, sometimes at the expense of employee well-being or customer satisfaction. In hospice care, it is essential that we remember our mission and ensure that metrics serve as a tool to enhance, rather than undermine, compassionate care.

I've observed that the most successful hospice organizations use metrics as a guide rather than a directive. Quality of care, patient satisfaction, and staff well-being remain the ultimate goals, and metrics are used to identify areas where improvements can support these goals. For instance, if patient satisfaction surveys reveal a need for better communication, the organization may invest in training programs to enhance staff-patient interactions. This approach ensures that metrics align with the organization's values and mission, fostering a culture that remains focused on compassionate, patient-centred care.

The Role of Continuous Improvement

In my corporate career, continuous improvement was a core principle, guiding organizations toward incremental changes that drive success. In hospice care, the philosophy of continuous improvement is equally important. By consistently assessing impact, gathering feedback, and analysing data, we can refine our practices, adapt to emerging needs, and enhance the quality of care we provide.

For example, many hospice organizations conduct regular reviews of patient outcomes and family satisfaction scores, using the findings to inform staff training, refine care protocols, and improve support services. Continuous improvement also involves staying informed about industry standards and best practices, incorporating insights from global benchmarks like the Quality of Death Index. This commitment to ongoing assessment and adjustment enables hospice organizations to meet the evolving needs of patients and families while upholding the highest standards of compassionate care.

Advocating for Quality Through Data

One of the most valuable lessons I've learned is the role of metrics in advocacy. In hospice care, data not only helps us assess our impact but also serves as a powerful tool for advocating change. Quantifiable metrics — such as patient satisfaction rates, symptom management outcomes, and accessibility statistics — provide a solid foundation for communicating the value of hospice care to policymakers, donors, and the public.

When advocating for regulatory changes or additional funding, data can make a compelling case. For example, by presenting statistics on the number of patients receiving pain relief, the organization can demonstrate the impact of improved medication access on patient comfort. Similarly, family satisfaction metrics can highlight the importance of end-of-life support, helping stakeholders understand the broader social and emotional benefits of hospice care.

In regions where palliative care is still developing, metrics play a crucial role in raising awareness and influencing policy. By demonstrating the tangible impact of hospice services, organizations can build support for their mission, secure funding, and advocate for the expansion of palliative care networks. Observing how data has transformed perceptions of palliative care around the world, particularly through frameworks like the Quality of Death Index, has reinforced my belief in the power of evidence-based advocacy.

Conclusion: Measuring What Matters

Measuring impact in hospice and palliative care requires a thoughtful balance between traditional metrics and mission-driven values. By focusing on quality, patient satisfaction, and operational efficiency, we can ensure that our services meet the highest standards of compassionate care. At the same time, we must remain mindful that our work is about people, not numbers. Metrics are simply a means to an end, helping us understand our strengths, address our challenges, and continue serving patients with dignity and respect.

As we move forward, the lessons learned from frameworks like the Quality of Death Index serve as a reminder of the importance of assessing impact on a broader scale. By measuring what matters, we can honour our mission, advocate for change, and contribute to a future where every person receives the compassionate end-of-life care they deserve.

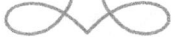

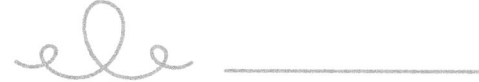

Chapter 10:
A Look Forward – Preparing for Future Challenges and Opportunities

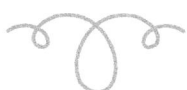

As I reach the end of this book, I am struck by how much I still have to learn. This journey into healthcare, especially hospice and palliative care has been both humbling and inspiring, and while I've shared what I've discovered along the way, I know there is still much I don't understand. The world of hospice and palliative care is complex, evolving, and deeply rooted in human experience – each patient, family member, and caregiver brings unique stories and needs. Writing this book has been my way of giving back, of advocating for a vision of sustainable, compassionate care that can meet the growing demands of an uncertain future.

Looking ahead, I see both challenges and opportunities in the field of hospice and palliative care. My hope is that the lessons I've shared here, drawn from my own journey and experiences, might serve as a guide or source of inspiration for others who are similarly invested in this work. This is not a comprehensive guide; rather, it's an account of my personal journey and what I have learned. As someone who came into this field as an amateur, I feel a profound responsibility to share my perspective, and I welcome others who wish to join me in learning, unlearning, and relearning. Let's make a difference together for a better world!

The Need for Adaptability in a Changing Healthcare Landscape

The future of hospice and palliative care will undoubtedly be shaped by a rapidly evolving healthcare landscape. Advances in technology, changing patient expectations, and shifting demographics are all influencing how care is delivered. The aging population in many parts of the world means that more people will need palliative and hospice care than ever before. Yet, the field itself is under-resourced, particularly in low- and middle-income countries where palliative care infrastructure is limited.

To meet these growing demands, hospice and palliative care must be adaptable and resilient. We will need to embrace technology thoughtfully, finding ways to integrate tools like telehealth, data analytics, and digital health records without losing the human connection that defines this work. Moreover, we must advocate for regulatory changes that support access to essential medications and pain relief, particularly in underserved areas. The goal is to build a hospice network that can thrive amidst these challenges, one that remains true to its mission of compassion while embracing innovation.

Embracing a Culture of Lifelong Learning

Entering this field from a corporate background, I quickly learned that hospice and palliative care is unlike any other type of work. Here, each day brings new experiences, insights, and lessons. I've had the privilege of learning from everyone around me – volunteers who give their time selflessly, patients who teach us about resilience and grace, and family caregivers who demonstrate remarkable strength and compassion. I often reflect on the words of Dame Cicely Saunders, the founder of modern palliative care:

"You matter because you are you, and you matter to the end of your life."

This quote has been a guiding light for me, reminding me of the deep respect and dignity that should underpin all hospice work. Saunders' words capture the essence of what makes hospice care unique: it is not about curing but about caring, about valuing each person as they are, in their most vulnerable moments. Her philosophy has influenced my philanthropic work and has been a constant source of inspiration as I work to build sustainable palliative care networks across the region. For me, this journey is a continuous cycle of learning, unlearning, and relearning – an ongoing commitment to honour the dignity of every individual we serve.

Future Challenges: Access, Funding, and Awareness

One of the most pressing challenges for the future of hospice and palliative care is access. In many countries, palliative care is still in its infancy, and large segments of the population lack access to even basic end-of-life support. Building sustainable hospice care networks in low-resource settings will require significant advocacy, education, and collaboration with local governments and healthcare providers. The Quality of Death Index has shown the stark disparities in palliative care access worldwide, and addressing these inequities must be a priority for all who work in this field.

Funding is another major challenge. Hospice care is resource-intensive, requiring specialized staff, medications, and facilities. As we look to the future, we must find innovative ways to secure sustainable funding — whether through public support, private donations, partnerships, or government subsidies. My experience in corporate finance has taught me the importance of revenue diversification, and I believe that hospice organizations must similarly embrace a range of funding sources to build resilience.

Public awareness is equally important. In many communities, misconceptions about hospice and palliative care persist, with some viewing it as "giving up" rather than as an opportunity for quality care at the end of life. Educating the public about the benefits of palliative care is essential, as is working with healthcare providers to encourage early referrals to hospice services. By promoting greater understanding and acceptance, we can ensure that more people benefit from compassionate end-of-life care.

Embracing Innovation While Staying True to Our Mission

As technology continues to advance, hospice care organizations will need to find ways to integrate new tools without sacrificing the human touch. Telehealth has already shown promise in expanding access to care, particularly in remote or underserved areas. Data analytics can help us better understand patient needs and optimize resource allocation. Digital health records can improve continuity of care and facilitate better communication between providers.

However, these innovations must be implemented carefully. Palliative care is, at its core, about connection and compassion. While technology can enhance certain aspects of care, it should never replace the face-to-face interactions that are so crucial in hospice work. Moving forward, we must ensure that innovation serves our mission and enhances, rather than detracts from, the personal connections that define hospice care.

A Vision for a Sustainable Hospice and Palliative Care Network

My vision for the future of palliative care is one of sustainability, compassion, and inclusivity. I believe in a model where hospice organizations work collaboratively with communities, healthcare providers, and governments to create systems of support that are accessible to all, regardless of income, geography, or cultural background. Sustainability means building networks that can endure economic pressures, adapt to changing healthcare landscapes, and continue providing high-quality, compassionate care to those in need.

As I reflect on this journey, I am deeply grateful for the lessons I've learned and the people who have guided me. This book is my way of giving back — a testament to the experiences, insights, and challenges I've encountered along the way. It is my hope that others, whether they are professionals in the field or newcomers drawn to the mission of hospice care, might find value in these pages.

Continuing the Journey

I am still learning, and I expect that I always will be. Hospice and palliative care is a field where no two days are alike, where each person brings something new to the table. Whether it's the wisdom of a volunteer, the courage of a patient, or the devotion of a family caregiver, there is always something to learn, unlearn, and relearn. This journey is not one that I walk alone; it is a collective effort,

Chapter 10: A Look Forward – Preparing for Future Challenges and Opportunities

supported by the dedication and compassion of countless individuals who believe in the value of end-of-life care.

In the words of Dame Cicely Saunders, "You matter because you are you, and you matter to the end of your life." As we move forward, I carry these words with me, a reminder of why we do this work and why it matters. The future of hospice care will bring challenges and change, but as long as we remain committed to the dignity, respect, and compassion that lie at the heart of our mission, we will continue to make a difference.

This book is not a definitive guide, nor is it an exhaustive exploration of hospice and palliative care. It is simply my story, my experiences, and my perspective. My hope is that it serves as a source of encouragement, a call to action, and a reminder of the profound importance of compassionate care. For those who choose to journey alongside me, whether as caregivers, advocates, or supporters, I extend my deepest gratitude. Together, we can build a future where hospice and palliative care is accessible, sustainable, and, above all, deeply compassionate.

A New Path: My Journey from Corporate into Hospice and Palliative Care Leadership

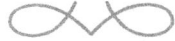

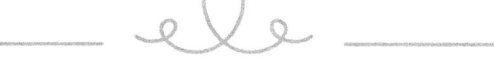

About the Author

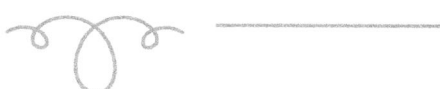

GIAM Cheong Leong, known to many simply as "Giam," transitioned into the world of hospice and palliative care after a successful career spanning over 20 years in corporate administration. With a background in strategic planning, financial management, and resource optimization, Giam initially built his expertise in high-stakes environments, managing substantial budgets and complex operations. However, a personal calling led him to explore a different kind of work — one focused not on profit margins but on compassion, community, and the dignity of life's final stages.

While Giam's journey into hospice and palliative care has been deeply fulfilling, he considers himself still an amateur in this field. His approach is one of openness and humility, learning from everyone around him, whether it be patients, caregivers, volunteers, or healthcare professionals. This work, he believes, requires continuous growth and reflection, and he is committed to sharing what he learns with those who may feel a similar calling.

Through this book, Giam hopes to inspire others — especially those with corporate backgrounds — to consider the unique and rewarding world of social healthcare. He believes that the skills cultivated in business settings, such as strategic thinking, management, and financial stewardship, can make a tremendous impact when applied to compassionate, patient-centred care. Giam welcomes like-minded individuals who wish to transition from corporate roles into social healthcare to connect, learn, and collaborate on meaningful, impactful work.

Giam's vision is to help build a network of compassionate, sustainable care that serves communities across the Asia Pacific region. His journey is a testament to the value of bringing diverse skills into new settings and a call for others to join him in making a difference. For those who share his passion for service, he extends an invitation to connect and explore the potential to transform lives through hospice and palliative care.

www.ingramcontent.com/pod-product-compliance
Lightning Source LLC
Chambersburg PA
CBHW050320230526
45471CB00005B/2280